LIVE LONGER

&

HEALTHIER

Discover the secrets of natural energies to live longer
and in good health.

1st edition

Volume 1

Jean Claude MEUX

~ 1 ~

VIVRE LONGTEMPS
& *EN*
BONNE SANTÉ

DÉCOUVRIR LES SECRETS DES ÉNERGIES NATURELLES
POUR VIVRE LONGTEMPS ET EN BONNE SANTÉ.

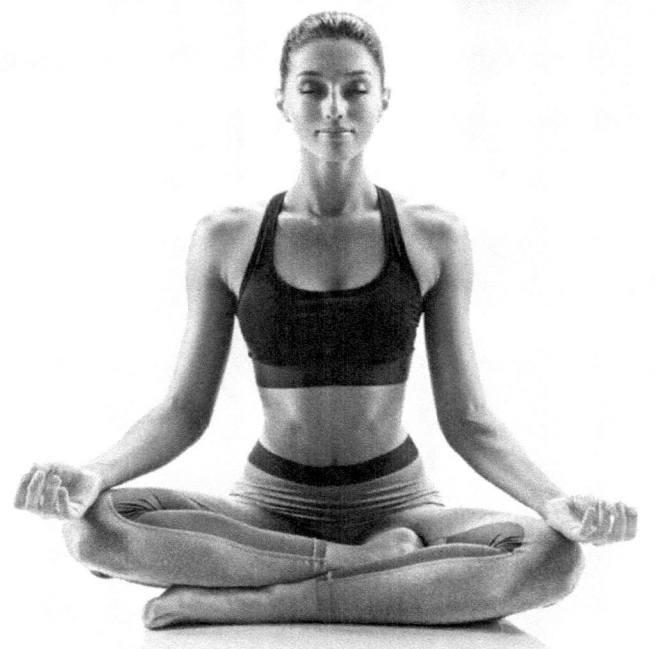

JEAN CLAUDE MEUX

LIVE LONGER

&

HEALTHIER

Discover the secrets of natural energies to live longer and in good health.

1st edition

Volume 1

Jean Claude MEUX

ISBN : 978-1-365-97291-1

ACKNOWLEDGEMENTS

A big thank you to Maxo LUCIEN that I contacted and who gave me some of his time for this collection.

All my thanks to Maxo LUCIEN Without him,

this collection would not have seen the day so quickly.

Website:

http://www.jcm.lu

FOREWORD

The world is moving. What shall I say? The world is moving at a dizzying speed from progress to progress. We don't even have time to get used to a new electronic gadget before another one replaces it. But it's not just in technology that things have changed a lot. Health and life quality are also changing. Important progress has been made in the healing and prevention of diseases and in life expectancy.

Who would have thought that you could live longer and still be healthy? And we are not presenting you with a science fiction novel where people can live almost forever and still stay young. We're being a little more realistic if we tell you that it is possible to slow down the aging process even though you're getting older, and still enjoy good health!

And who knows ? With the development of modern medicine, in the centuries or even decades to come, perhaps man will be able to overcome aging and achieve immortality. But for now, let us present you this guide that shows you how to combine old age, youth and health.

Table des matières

The Guide To Your Wellness!

INTRODUCTION

Would you like to live a long and healthy life?

Wanting to live longer is a great goal. But gaining extra years doesn't mean much if they can't be lived in health and energy. So why not at the same time allow your body to run in a healthy way that is younger than your chronological age? It's not difficult. All you have to do is apply the methods and principles we will reveal in this book. Just as some practices can deteriorate your health and reduce your life expectancy. Others, on the other hand, can improve your body and help you live longer. Such practices not only extend your life span, but also improve the quality of your health by protecting your body from diseases.

You will discover step by step these methods to make your life better and to live longer and healthier.

STAYING YOUNG AND HEALTHY IS POSSIBLE.

Improved living conditions and medical advances over the past 50 years have extended current life expectancy to around 20 years and probably beyond 90 or 100 for future generations.

Did you know that it is possible to live beyond 125 years, in a healthy and rejuvenated body? This is not a wild claim to get attention or to sell a product, but a goal that each of us can set and achieve without difficulty. It is legitimate to want to live longer and in perfect health. And the best part is that it is possible and within reach for all of us.

The component related to this phenomenon is the telomere. A telomere is a repeating region located at the end of our chromosomes. This region tends to shorten with age, inflammation and stress. Studies have shown that short telomeres are associated with a higher risk of age-related diseases. Therefore, a lack of telomeres would mean the rapid loss of genetic information necessary for cell function. The good news is that 2009 Nobel Prize-winning scientist Elizabeth Blackburn discovered what is called telomerase. That is, a process that allows the cell to regenerate.

that is to say a process that allows to lengthen the size of telomeres, thus the life span.

On the other hand, in a study published on January 8 in the BMJ, it is revealed that a healthy lifestyle can indeed contribute to increasing the number of years of life without disease. The results of this study show that women can extend their disease-free life expectancy after age 50 by about 10 years, and men by about 8 years more, compared to people who do not have these habits...

A HEALTHY AND REJUVENATING DIET

It is no longer proven that the food we eat has a considerable impact on the state of our health. That's why having a healthy body inevitably requires a healthy, appropriate and balanced diet. But food can also play other roles, such as keeping our bodies young.

1. A balanced diet

Among the balanced diets we find mainly the Mediterranean diet, the DASH diet and the MIND diet...

a. The Mediterranean diet

The Mediterranean diet is perfect for fighting cholesterol problems. It reduces bad cholesterol while promoting good cholesterol. In addition, this diet helps reduce the risk of heart disease, stroke, type 2 diabetes and cancer. It is a diet that is rich in cereals, vegetables, legumes, fish, foods containing antioxidants, etc. In addition, it helps to fight brain aging.

b. The DASH diet

The DASH (Dietary Approaches to Stopping Hypertension) diet is mainly based on nutrients that are related to blood pressure such as sodium, calcium and potassium. This is why this diet is very effective in lowering blood pressure. The DASH diet consists of vegetables, fruits, grain

grain products, low-fat or fat-free dairy products, lean meat, poultry, fish, nuts, seeds and dried beans

c. The MIND diet

MIND is an acronym that stands for Mediterranean-DASH Intervention for Neurodegenerative Delay. In general, it improves health. But more specifically it serves as a prevention against cognitive decline and Alzheimer's disease. It is a diet that is designed to ensure the proper functioning of the brain. The foods that make up this diet are good fats or lipids rich in Omega-3, green leafy vegetables, seafood, fruits, etc. Water is also an extremely important element in this diet.

2. Les nutrients

Vitamins and minerals are extremely important for the body. You must consume them in sufficient quantities and in a varied manner. They are even more necessary for people aged 50 and over. Try to consume the following main nutrients.

a. B12 vitamins

With age, our body's ability to absorb B12 vitamin gradually decreases. This is why it is important to ensure that we consume enough of it. Because a deficiency in this vitamin can have harmful effects on the body such as tiredness, paleness, unusual muscle weakness, shortness of breath, memory problems, palpitations, nausea and digestive problems. You will find B12 vitamin in red meat, white meat, offal, eggs, salmon, tuna, clams, sardines, mackerel, trout, oysters, mussels, milk, Emmental cheese and Camembert cheese.

b. D vitamin

D vitamin has several functions in the body: it allows us to absorb calcium. This helps us to keep our bones healthy and ensures the proper functioning of our nerves and the strengthening of our immune system.

c. E Vitamin

E Vitamin helps to fight cataracts. Yes, antioxidants such as lutein or zeaxanthin, contained in egg yolks, spinach and other green vegetables, could reduce the risk of contracting a cataract. It is important to eat foods containing this vitamin. It is also found in nuts. Be sure to eat 1/4 cup of nuts a day. Also, E vitamin is an antioxidant that plays a huge role in immune system function.

d. Manganese

Manganese is essential for the action of enzymes. Without it, enzymes cannot do their work in the body. Manganese contributes to the metabolism of sugars and to the synthesis of lipids in men (male sex). The main foods that contain manganese are mussels, hazelnuts, pumpkin seeds, wheat bran muffin, oatmeal, brown rice, cereals, multigrain, beans, whole wheat pasta, pineapple, whole grain bread, oysters, firm tofu, brewed tea, fresh soybeans (edamame), quinoa, chocolate, raspberries, raw spinach.

e. Potassium

As we get older, we have difficulty moving our muscles. So, you should know that potassium is extremely important for muscle contraction. This nutrient is found in meat, beans, dried fruits, fish, flaxseed, garlic, bananas, avocados, sweet potatoes, potatoes, etc.

f. Les proteins

Sarcopenia is when our muscles lose strength. This phenomenon is established in our body as we get older. We can always do exercises to strengthen our muscles but we can also consume proteins. Proteins are a guarantee for strong muscles. Protein is found in meat, fish, milk, almonds, shrimp, lentils, parmesan cheese, salmon, soybeans, tuna, legumes, grains and oilseeds.

BEST PRACTICES TO STAY YOUNG AND KEEP HEALTHY.

Staying young is the dream of all of us, yet we do not know how to achieve this goal. So, in this section we reveal some practices that if you apply them and without having to change your habits too much, you can gain more than 25 years of healthy life compared to someone who does not follow them.

1. A 6-point method for a young and healthy body.

a. Avoid smoking and drink a bit of alcohol

Tobacco is the most important pro-geriatric factor. In addition, it can cause more than twenty chronic diseases such as stroke, vision loss, cataract, age-related macular degeneration, periodontitis, asthma, pneumonia, thoracic aortic aneurysm, peripheral arterial disease, atherosclerosis, diabetes, effects on the female reproductive system, erectile dysfunction, birth defect, immune deficiency, etc.

Although a little of alcohol is good for the body, heavy drinking has devastating effects on our health. It causes short-term discomfort and long-term illnesses. In the short term, alcohol acts as a sedative that makes us drowsy, impairs our coordination, causes alertness problems and can even cause an alcoholic coma. In the long term, alcohol consumption carries the risk of serious diseases such as cancer, diseases of the nervous and mental systems, cancers and cirrhosis.

b. Choose a normal weight

It is important to have a normal weight or rather to have what we call a healthy weight. That is, a weight that does not pose a risk to our health. This weight is not the same for everyone. It varies from one person to another. It depends on our body mass index (BMI). But we do not all have the same BMI. In any case, it is absolutely necessary to avoid overweight and obesity. Because they carry serious risks for our health. Indeed, they can cause cardiovascular diseases, cancers, high blood pressure, respiratory difficulties, etc.

A healthy diet for a young and healthy body. It is essential to eat foods that are not only safe for the body but also necessary for its proper functioning. This is a must. You can't want to preserve your health and eat anything at the same time. You have to eat healthy meals. An example of a healthy meal includes vegetables, fruits and small portions of protein and whole grains. These foods provide fiber and important nutrients such as vitamins and minerals. When planning meals for you and your family, consider including.

Foods to prioritize are salads or other vegetables of different colors, such as spinach, sweet potatoes and red, green, orange or yellow peppers, fat-free or low-fat milk and dairy products, or non-dairy products such as almond or rice milk, different colored fruits such as apples, bananas and grapes, lean beef or pork or other protein foods such as chicken, seafood, eggs, tofu or beans, whole grains such as brown rice, oatmeal, whole grain bread and whole grain cornmeal.

Sweets are acceptable as long as they are not eaten regularly. You should only touch them occasionally. It is not acceptable to eat candy, ice cream or cookies on a daily basis. Limit these sweet treats to special occasions, and take small portions. Avoid buying single servings of pizza slices from snack bars, industrialized or prepared foods.

Don't forget milk. It is a good source of calcium and protein and is rich in A, B1 and B2 Vitamin. But if you are lactose intolerant, meaning that you have trouble digesting the sugar in milk, then you can try lactose-free milk or yogurt. In addition to milk and dairy products, you can get calcium from calcium-fortified cereals, fruit juices and soy or nut drinks. Eating dark green leafy vegetables, such as kale and collards, and soft-boned canned fish, such as salmon, can also help you meet your body's calcium needs.

Try dried beans, such as black beans, butter beans, kidney beans and others. They are high in protein, less expensive and a quick and easy addition to your meals. Eat fatty fish like salmon, mackerel, herring and tuna. They are the best source of omega-3 essential fatty acids that protect the body against cardiovascular disease (especially in combination with statins), type II diabetes and rheumatoid arthritis. Choose foods rich in antioxidants, which can slow down the aging process of the body and brain.

d. Exercice or practice sport

Sports or exercise are important to reduce your risk of developing chronic diseases such as heart disease, diabetes and obesity. You can do them at least 2 to 3 times a week. It doesn't have to be competitive, just 10 to 20 minutes of biking or walking, for example, will boost your energy levels and get rid of any signs of tiredness.

Whether it's pushing back bedtime to meet a deadline or missing a few hours of sleep due to work schedules, many people cut back on the hours they should be spending in bed. As a result, 15-35% of the general population is sleep deprived, depriving them of vital rest time. This lack of sleep is not without consequences on our health. It can make you feel lethargic, cranky and tired. If you often feel this way, you should ask yourself if you are getting enough sleep. If the answer is no, then your remedy may simply be good, long sleep.

It is actually recommended that you get about 7 hours of sleep per night, although some people need a little more and some need a little less. If you are not getting as much sleep as you need, you can try to relax before bed. You

You can take a bath, read a book or go to bed a half hour earlier than usual.

SOCIAL CONNECTIONS FOR BETTER HEALTH

One of the most important factors in establishing a longevity lifestyle is belonging to a broader social network, in addition to the support of friends and family. In fact, scientific research has shown that staying connected and integrated into one's community is one of the strongest predictors of greater longevity.

According to a U.S. government study, social isolation promotes declining mental function in older adults. It is strongly advised to set aside time in your life for shared activities and to make sure you have expanded your network as widely as possible. And in some moments when you will be alone you can indulge in games such as crossword puzzles, sudoku, instead of taking your head with anxious thoughts.

However, if you find that the members of your social circle do not share your values and aspirations, then you just have to choose your team. In this case, you will select a few friends and confidants with whom you can share great moments and who can help you through difficult times. This will help you strengthen your immune system and thus keep you healthy.

1. Stress management

People who are very diligent about diet and exercise may overlook the impact of stress on their health. Stress has many physiological effects, including an increase in cortisol levels. Cortisol is a hormone secreted by our body under the effect of stress. It can cause cardiovascular problems, dangerous abdominal fat, depression and lower resistance to disease.

Stress can mean difficulty to stay focus, racing thoughts and difficulty disconnecting. It can affect anyone. In fact, even people with busy lives can feel stressed, anxious or overwhelmed. This can have a negative impact on your physical and mental health.

But don't panic! We're not giving you all this information about stress to freak you out. That's why we also offer you ways to avoid and escape stress. It's all about minimizing lifestyle stress in order to increase your energy levels. Strategies to do this include taking time to relax, read or take a walk. As a bonus, you'll find the secrets to getting the upper hand on stress in this ebook.

2. Connect with nature

With an increasingly busy lifestyle, many people regularly feel tired and run down. However, if the tiredness you feel is related to your lifestyle, there are many activities you can do to increase your natural energy level and improve your life.

3. The energies of nature

Nature is an inexhaustible source of natural energies. You can use its energies intelligently to make your life easier and richer. Take time to embrace nature, alone, with family or friends.

Staying close to nature can only be beneficial to your health. For example, outdoor activities reduce the risk of developing vision problems like farsightedness and nearsightedness. A study of children in Australia found that school-aged children who participated in outdoor activities had better vision than those who spent more time indoors.

This study is also true with the multiplication of electronic games and video game consoles that confirm this approach. After reading these tips, change your habits if you were not in that population of people who ignore the benefits that nature can bring them.

4. Nature as a source of energy treatment

Nature walks are beneficial for people with depression. Studies have shown that people with this disorder have experienced significant improvements in their mood when exposed to nature. They feel more motivated and energetic to recover and return to normal. In addition, walking in nature and the outdoors reduces stress by lowering cortisol (the stress hormone) in the body.

Walking in a natural environment has positive impacts not only on our physical health but also on our mental health. Indeed, this walk is beneficial for the heart, the muscles and the general metabolism. And scientists have proven that walking in nature also improves our emotional health.

A study conducted and published by Stanford University in California found that participants who walked in green parks demonstrated increased attention and focus, more so than participants who walked in enclosed urban environments.

The exact mechanism by which nature helps mood disorders is unclear, but researchers agree that, time spent in nature tends to lift mood. Indeed, when they are exposed even briefly to nature, people's moods improve. It appears that high levels of negative ions in the air near moving water, a forest or a mountain potentially reduce symptoms of depression

STAY CONNECTED WITH NATURE

1. Spend 20 minutes a day in nature.

Commit to spending 20 minutes a day in nature. You can use this time by hiking, walking, gardening, sitting or meditating. Whatever you choose to do, do it with full awareness. Use all your senses, observe your surroundings without judgment, and enjoy whatever surrounds you that brings your body and mind into a state of calm.

2. Splurge with plants.

Put a houseplant in your office or other areas where you spend a lot of time. The sight of plants and greenery has been shown to help improve attention and even decrease pain. One study found that placing a plant in a hospital room reduces the length of hospital stay, the need for pain medication and the negative comments nurses write in patients' charts.

3. Find a room with a nature view

Some studies have shown that people heal faster in the hospital and have more energy at work when they have a view of nature rather than a built environment. If possible, try to spend most of your time at home or in a room that offers a view of greenery. If this is not possible, you can hang pictures or paintings of nature in your view. You can also choose as your wallpaper or screensaver on your smartphone or computer or tablet a picture of nature.

4. Make it a retreat.

Getting away, relaxing and spending time in nature by meditating, eating healthy and sleeping deeply is a great way to rest, renew and get back on track. According to a recent study published in the Journal of Psychosomatic Research, meditation retreats are moderately effective in reducing anxiety, depression and stress and improving quality of life.

5. Connect to nature though food

This one is a bit obvious, but if it doesn't come from the earth, your body won't respond well to it. Think about bringing nature into your body, especially if you can't get out into nature regularly. Eat foods that are naturally available on this earth and shop in the outer reaches of the grocery store, buying vegetables, fruits, nuts and seeds, lean and hormone-free proteins, and healthy grains. Better yet, plant your own vegetables if you can. You

You'll get the combined benefits of healthy eating and being in nature.

THE HEALTH BENEFITS OF NATURE

1. It stimulates the mood

Going outside in the warmth of a sunny day is a great way to bring a smile to your face. And there's a reason for that. Sunlight gives you nourishing and energizing D vitamin. It's been shown to improve mood, calm the nervous system and improve problems such as seasonal depression.

In addition, D vitamin also promotes the absorption of calcium in the body, minimizes the risk of high blood pressure, cancer and certain autoimmune diseases.

2. It allows you to stay in the present

Disconnecting from everyday life and getting outdoors allows you to focus on the present moment. In essence, contact with nature encourages you to be in the "here and now", calming your mind and helping you enjoy the sights, sounds and smells that surround you but that you may not have noticed.

It is a basic form of meditation that helps reduce stress and anxiety by focusing your attention on the present moment instead of dwelling on bad memories or worrying about an uncertain future.

3. It gives you energy

You may think a double espresso is the key to overcoming an afternoon slump, but research suggests that a walk in the woods is more effective. A series of studies published in the Journal of Environmental Psychology found that people who were exposed to nature for just 20 minutes a day had higher energy levels and a better overall mood than those who were not.

.

4. Nature can make you a good person

A University of Rochester study found that people exposed to nature tend to feel more generous, more connected to their community, and more socially conscious. Simply looking at pictures of nature reinforces feelings of connection with other living things. It reminds us of core values such as generosity and caring..

5. Nature strengthens your spirituality

Connecting with nature can have a deeply spiritual side, helping to strengthen our sense of spiritual or divine identity. We may be part of a larger universe than we can imagine, but that doesn't mean we can't find comfort in the vast environment around us. surrounding us. Reconnect by doing something as simple as walking barefoot on the mossy forest floor or dipping your toes in the ocean.

6. How to get your daily dose of nature?

Making a conscious decision to bring more nature into your life is the first step to taking advantage of its healing powers. Spend time planting in your garden or simply relaxing in your yard. Try leaving your phone, tablet or book inside and instead focus on the smells, sounds, sights and textures around you - the scent of your rose garden, the feel of the wind on your face, the song of the birds. When it's time to return to your regular activities, remember that even managing life can often be done outside; paying a few bills from your patio, for example.

Also try to exercise outdoors. Do your morning yoga in a park or take a walk on a nature trail instead of the treadmill. Nourish your body and soul by dining outside at office lunch or family dinner.

If you can't spend as much time outside as you'd like, bring a touch of the outdoors inside. Add indoor plants to your home or office, or even an office water fountain. The sound of running water can have a calming effect, and studies have shown that indoor plants can reduce headaches and fatigue

LET'S RECAP: TECHNICAL KEY FOR LIVING LONGER AND HEALTHIER

This guide gives you the top secrets to staying healthy. You have the power to change many things that can affect your well-being and the length of your life. Here is a summary of 10 steps you can take to help you live the longest and healthiest life possible:

Do not smoke.

- Get regular physical activity, stay active every day.

- Eat a healthy diet rich in whole grains, lean protein, vegetables and fruit. Reduce or avoid saturated and unhealthy trans fats. Choose healthier monounsaturated and polyunsaturated fats instead.

- See your doctor regularly.

- Make sure you get enough D vitamin and calcium.

- Maintain a healthy weight and body type.

- Challenge your mind (memory games, sudoku, word searches, etc.)

- Build a strong social network.

- Protect your sight, hearing and overall health by following preventive care guidelines.

- Get enough sleep.

3 BONUS AS A CONCLUSION

1. Discover and learn continously

a. Intellectual growth

Learning helps us live longer and healthier lives. These benefits are numerous. Indeed, learning allows for the stimulation of brain connections, relaxation, less stress, relief from chronic pain, a good mood, protection for cognitive functions, etc.

According to a study conducted in India, reading is capable of developing the brain. In fact, people who learn to read in their thirties show changes in the regions of the brain that manage motor skills, vision and hearing. An American study has even shown that diligent reading can contribute to prolonging our life expectancy.

The simple fact of investing a total of 3h30 in reading per week can protect the brain from regenerative diseases. Reading would therefore be a good way to preserve our cognitive abilities even as we age.

In this study, Professor Becca Levy noted that "people who read even a little, even half an hour a day, had a significant survival advantage over those who did not read".

Intellectual stimulation in later life has been shown to have significant health benefits for seniors. According to Simon Fraser University, learning strengthens the immune system of seniors. It also makes them less anxious and less socially isolated..

b. Borad games

Board games are well known for their ability to create and strengthen social bonds. However, they have other virtues that are just as interesting. They prove to be a good way to prevent health problems. They help preserve the memory of the elderly. They also help slow down Alzheimer's disease. Playing board games means having fun while improving your mental health.

It may sound incredible, but it's scientifically proven that traveling keeps you young and healthy. This was shown in a study conducted by the **Transamerica Center for Retirement Studies**. Traveling has a variety of benefits for both physical and mental health. According to the **Framingham Heart Study Research Institute** in Massachusetts, "*going on vacation regularly reduces cardiovascular risks by 30%*". This is because the novelty can provoke the production of adrenaline, a hormone that is very beneficial for the heart. This is how travel reduces the risk of heart disease. When you are immersed in a new environment, it causes an increase in neurons. This makes the brain more efficient. Because it is stimulated.

2. Think positively.

a. Staying optimistic

Yes, we know that evil exists. But if we focus on the good aspects of things, the bad ones will not have any influence on us. Because things only have the importance that we give them. The question is then to know what is really important to you. Your fears or your dreams? Your misadventures or your achievements?

Say goodbye to your fears and head straight for your happiness. Smile at life and it will smile back at you. Stop experiencing life as a burden or punishment and enjoy it instead as a delicious dish.

See nature, see how wonderful it is! Realize that it offers you everything you need to live. Be aware of all the good things it has to offer. And stop adding to it the evils you fear. These fears, these anxieties could only harm your physical health as well as your mental health. All this stress that you are poisoning yourself with will eventually cause your premature aging.

La Bruyère wrote that *"the spirit of politeness is a attention to make others happy with us by our words and manners"*. Indeed, to be courteous is to make sure that one's presence is a source of well-being for others, so as not to unfairly infringe on the physical integrity, dignity and modesty of others.

Apply the golden rule in your relationships with others. According to this rule, you should not do to others what you would not want done to you or your loved ones. The benefits of these principles are enormous and very beneficial in your life. It leaves you on good terms with others. This avoids a lot of annoyance that could affect your health and cause you worry.

However, it can happen to you to be prejudicial to the others without wanting it and without you knowing it but simply because you do not master the rules of good manners. So, to avoid such inconveniences you can get books dealing with the question of good manners. But in the meantime, we give you these little magic words: Hello, goodbye, please, thank you, sorry, etc. It seems basic, even banal. And yet many conflicts and difficulties could have been avoided if the people involved had simply used these magic words

had simply used these magic words at the right moment. Apply them every time the opportunity arises and you will notice the difference in your daily life

c. Be grateful

It may not seem obvious, but being grateful for the little things in life is a great service we can do for ourselves. It not only helps us to bear life with more joy and tranquility, but also allows us to benefit from the big things.

It's simple, "*energy flows where attention goes*" as Rhonda Byrne points out in The Secret. So, the more you focus on what's going well in your life, the more you give yourself the chance to improve what's not.

3. Get rid of stress

As we have seen above, stress is a disease-causing factor and promotes premature aging.

That is why it is necessary to get rid of it or learn to manage it. To do this, you can use the following principles and practices.

- Get enough sleep

- Get physical exercise

- Have a fulfilling social life

- Do some reading

- Meditate a little

- Entertain yourself: music, movies, theater, dance, games, etc.

- Laugh as often as possible: watch funny videos or read jokes, joke with friends

- Organize yourself better. Sometimes it is the lack of discipline in daily activities that causes stress.

- Take a walk. Ideally, you should go for a walk in nature, in the middle of a forest, river and birds

Official website:

www.jcm.lu

September 2021

TIPS :

New tips are updated on the editor's website: don't hesitate to visit it from time to time. A newsletter is there to be informed first.

A question, a problem ...

Visit the website, contact information is available.

Official website:

www.jcm.lu

Mail contact :

contact@jcm.lu